MEDICAL HOUSESTAFF
SURVIVAL GUIDE
"MODI'S PRACTICAL PEARLS"

DR. ANANG MODI

2ND EDITION

ISBN: 1468009494
ISBN 13: 9781468009491

TABLE OF CONTENTS

INTRODUCTION:

Four years of college, four years of medical school and you start your first day of residency only to realize just how much more there is still to learn. Your pager is constantly beeping as you are being bombarded with questions that you feel seem simple but yet are not confident enough to answer. You completed four challenging years of medical school and you passed all your board exams and are a now finally a physician but you are not sure how to write an order, supplement potassium or what to do when a patient is short of breath. You want to ask your resident but know that they are also extremely busy and you feel uncomfortable paging the attending directly for every minor issue. "Modi's Practical Pearls" is a quick, handy, reference book that can help guide you through almost any issue encountered on the medical wards and ICU. It was written by me as a senior resident and given to my interns. They loved it so much that it was given to the entire intern class and now has been given to every single medicine intern at Winthrop University Hospital for the last seven years. It is also great for physician assistants, nurse practitioners, medical and PA students and almost any healthcare professional. They all have found it to be very helpful in managing day to day problems encountered on the medical wards and ICU. After years of encouraging me to write a book, I decided to share these pearls with all of you and published Medical Housestaff Survival Guide: Modi's Practical Pearl in 2006. Now I am updating and improving this book in this new 2nd Edition.

I would like to dedicate this book to my wife, Vinita, for all her love and support and for being such a wonderful physician, companion and best friend. I would also like to dedicate this book to all the interns, residents, PA's, N.P.'s, medical students and housestaff for their endless hours of hard work and unrelenting passion to help others.

Anang Modi

Note to the reader: Although the information in this book has been carefully reviewed, neither the author nor the editor or publisher can accept any legal responsibility for any errors or omissions. The contents of this book are merely guidelines and do not substitute for a particular clinical scenario. Application of this material to a particular situation remains the professional responsibility of the practitioner. Readers are encouraged to confirm the information contained in this book with other sources. Before prescribing any drug the reader should review the manufacturer's current product information, correct dosages, and accepted indications.

COMMON PROBLEMS
ON THE MEDICAL WARDS:

Electrolyte abnormalities:

Potassium (K) disroders: (normal K = 3.6-5.0 mmol/L)

Hypokalemia:
- Common causes of hypokalemia in the hospital include: Diarrhea, medications (<u>diuretics</u>, insulin, beta-2 agonists), type 1 & type 2 renal tubular acidosis (RTA), hypomagnesemia, alkalosis and mineralcorticoid excess.
- Potassium (K) can be supplemented po (by mouth) or IV.
- K-Dur (pill) comes in 20 mEq and 40 mEq po
- K-Lor (liquid) also comes in 20mEq and 40 mEq p
- When supplementing potassium orally or IV remember that for every 10 mEq you give, it should increase the K by about 0.1 (thus if the K is 3.5 you can give K-Dur 40 mEq po x 1 and it should increase the K to 3.9 in healthy patients)
- You can't give more than 40 mEq over a 4 hour period. Therefore, if a patient's potassium is 3.1, then you can give K-Dur 40 mEq po x 1 now and then give K-Dur 20 mEq four hours later.
- If the pt is npo (nothing by mouth) and needs supplementation then you can give potassium chloride (KCL) as 10 mEq in 100cc's of sterile water x 1 or 2 runs each to run over 1 hour (you can give up to a maximum of 3 runs). Each 10mEq IV run of KCL should raise the potassium by about 0.1 as well.

- Each IV KCL run should be given over one hour. You should not give more than 3 consecutive runs. If you need to give more, repeat a K level 4 hours after the last run and then you can supplement more if needed.
- In a patient that is running a persistently low K that is on IVF you can also add K to the IVF. This has to be done with caution since it may be easy to forget that the patient is getting K in the IVF and this may lead to hyperkalemia. Also, a covering house officer may get called for a slightly low potassium and decide to supplement po or IV over the phone without the nurse or house officer realizing that the patient is already on potassium in the IVF bag. This may lead to over-supplementation.
- If you need to recheck the potassium later that day then do it 4 hours after the last IV run or 4 hours after the last po dose to allow time for equilibration.

Cautions:

- Be <u>extremely cautious</u> in supplementing K in patients with renal insufficiency as they tend to retain K and are at risk for developing hyperkalemia. Hyperkalemia can lead to serious arrythmias.
- Do not give more than 40 mEq of K within a span of 4 hours
- Make sure the patient has good IV access when giving IV KCL.

Practical Pearls:

- If a patient has a low K that is not rising as expected, check the magnesium (Mg) since a low Mg will cause the potassium to remain low even despite supplementation.

- When addressing a low K, you should always try to figure out the reason why the patient is hypokalemic and try to address this as well.

Hyperkalemia:

- Common causes of hyperkalemia in the hospital include: Renal failure, medications (K sparing diuretics, ACE inhibitors, NSAID's, beta-blockers), acidosis, hypoaldosteronism/ adrenal insufficiency, rhabdomyolysis, iatrogenic, and pseudo-hyperkalemia (hemolysis, marked leukocytosis).
- If the K is greater than 5.6 or if the patient is symptomatic it is a good idea to check an EKG to check for any changes from hyperkalemia (peaked T waves, wide QRS).
- If you suspect EKG changes from hyperkalemia (such as peaked T waves) then you need to give calcium chloride or calcium gluconate stat to prevent any arrhythmia. *Note:* calcium will not lower the K, it only decreases membrane excitability and temporarily decreases the chances of hyperkalemia induced arrhythmias.
- If the K is <u>unexpectedly</u> elevated and the patient is <u>asymptomatic</u>, you should repeat the K stat (may be hemolyzed or lab error giving a falsely elevated K)
- If hyperkalemia is real, then give 8-10 units of insulin with 1-2 amps of D50 (to prevent hypoglycemia from the insulin). *Note:* check an accu-check before the insulin because if the glucose is very high you may not need to give the D50.
- In addition to the above, you can also give Albuterol treatment (beta- 2 agonists can lower K) or Lasix (if no contra-indications) to lower the potassium.

- *Note:* Insulin and albuterol just make the K go from extra to intracellular and thus their effects are temporary.
- Kayexalate should be given, in addition to the above, to rid the body of potassium. The potassium will not go down until the patient has a bowel movement from the Kayexalate. *Note:* Kayexalate will give the patient diarrhea.
- Kayexalate can be given as 15 grams or 30 grams po x 1.
- If the K is not dangerously high and the patient is <u>asymptomatic</u> then you can treat with Kayexalate alone.
- You should repeat the potassium later on in the day to confirm that the K has come down.

Practical Pearls:
- In a patient with significant hyperkalemia it is always a good idea to check an EKG, even if they are asymptomatic.
- In a patient with renal failure, significant hyperkalemia is an indication for urgent dialysis.

Magnesium (Mg) Disorders:
(Normal Mg =1.5-2.2 mEq/L)

Hypomagnesemia:

- Common causes of low magnesium include: Malabsorption, diarrhea, diuretics, alcoholism and hypercalcemia
- Treatment of low Mg:
  - » For mild hypomagnesemia you can give Mag-oxide 400mg po bid x 1-2 days
  - » For moderate hypomagnesemia or if the patient is npo you can give Mag-sulfate 1 gram or 2 grams in 100cc NS (normal saline) x 1 run.

Practical Pearls:

- A chronically low Mg will also result in a low K and a low Ca.
- Mag-oxide may cause some diarrhea.

Phosphorus (Phos) Disorders:
(Normal Phos = 3.0-4.5 mg/dl)

Phosphorus (Ph):

- Common causes of hypophosphatemia include: Alcohol abuse, hyperparathyroidism, malabsorption, oral phosphate binders, DKA, vitamin D deficiency, glucose infusion, Fanconi's syndrome and hyperalimentation.
- Treatment of low phos:
  - » If mild hypophosphatemia you can supplement with neutra-phos 2 packets po bid x 1 day. Note: this often gives the patient diarrhea.
  - » For more severe hypophosphatemia you can give phosphorus IV as sodium-phos (Na-phos) 10 mEq in 100cc NS (normal saline) x 1 or 2 runs.
  - » If the patient has a low K and a low phosphorus, then you can give K-Phos 10 mEq in 100cc's NS x 1 or 2 runs, each to run over 1 hour.

Practical Pearl:

- Be extremely cautious in supplementing phosphorus in a renal patient since they retain phosphorus and can easily become hyper-phosphatemic.

Calcium (Ca) Disorders: (Normal Ca = 8.6-10.3 mg/dl)

Hypocalcemia:

- Common causes of hypocalcemia include: Hypoparathyroidism, renal failure, acute pancreatitis, malabsorption, rhabdomyolysis, hyper and hypomagnesemia, vitamin D deficiency, medications and multiple citrated blood transfusions
- Treatment:
    - » Can supplement orally with calcium carbonate as 1500 mg po 2-3 times a day for 1-3 days for mild asymptomatic hypocalcemia.
    - » Severe, symptomatic hypocalcemia can be treated with calcium gluconate IV.

Practical Pearl:

- A common cause of a "falsely" low serum calcium is hypoalbuminemia. Before supplementing the calcium calculate the corrected calcium. This is done by simply adding 0.8 mg/dl to the calcium for every 1 g/dl decrease in serum albumin from 4.0 g/dl. For example, if a patient has a serum calcium of 8.0 and a serum albumin of 3.0, then the corrected calcium is really 8.8 and falls within the normal range and the patient does not need calcium supplementation.

Hypercalcemia:

- Common causes of hypercalcemia include: Hyperparathyroidism, myeloma, malignancy/ metastases, addison's, sarcoidosis, hyperthyroidism, milk-alkali, vitamin D intoxication, thiazides, lithium and immobilization.
- Symptoms of hypercalcemia can include abdominal pain, constipation, nausea, weakness, confusion/ stupor, polyuria, arrythmia (short QT interval).

- Hypercalcemia can also cause pancreatitis, diabetes insipidus and kidney stones.
- Treatment:
  - » In a symptomatic patient or a patient with a very high calcium (≥12mg/dl) treat with normal saline.
  - » <u>After the patient has been well hydrated with normal saline</u>, you can give furosemide at 20-40mg IV bid (if no contraindications).
  - » In a patient with severe hypercalcemia pamidronate can also be given. However, the response is not seen acutely and can take a few days.
  - » Calcitonin lowers serum calcium within a few hours and can be used early in the treatment of severe hypercalcemia along with saline and furosemide.
- In patients with severe hypercalcemia that are not responding to medical therapy or with contraindications to IVF hydration, hemodialysis should be considered.

Sodium (Na) Disorders: (Normal Na = 135-145 mmol/L)

Hyponatremia:

- Common causes of hyponatremia in the hospital include: CHF/fluid overload, cirrhosis, hyperglycemia, SIADH, renal insufficiency, diuretic use, hypoaldosteronism, vomiting, polydipsia, adrenal insufficiency, and hypothyroidism.
- The approach to a patient with hyponatremia should initially focus on 2 main aspects: serum osmolality (S osm) and volume status.
- If the S osm is high (> 295 mosm/kg) and the patient is hyponatremic then you should look into causes such as hyperglycemia, mannitol and radiocontrast agents.
- If the S osm is normal with hyponatremia then you should look for paraproteinemia or hyperlipidemia (high triglycerides).
- If the serum osm is low then you should assess ECF (extracellular fluid) volume:
- If the ECF volume is increased: rule out causes such as CHF, cirrhosis, nephrotic syndrome or renal insufficiency.
- If the ECF volume is normal: rule out SIADH, hypothyroidism, psychogenic polydipsia and adrenal insufficiency.
- If the ECF is decreased then you should check a urine Na concentration:
  - » If urine Na is < 10mmol/L then the hyponatremia may be from vomiting, diuretics or diarrhea.
  - » If urine Na is > 20mmol/L then the hyponatremia may be from salt wasting, hypoaldosteronism, diuretics or ACE inhibitors.

- Treatment of hyponatremia:
  - » If symptomatic hyponatremia (confusion, mental status changes, seizures) then you need to treat with hypertonic 3% saline with furosemide in an ICU setting. Careful and frequent monitoring of Na is necessary to avoid an overly rapid correction of sodium since this may precipitate central pontine myelinolysis. Plasma Na should not be raised by more than 10mmol/L during the first 24 hours.
  - » For asymptomatic hypotonic, hypovolemic hyponatremia treatment is to give Normal Saline.
  - » For asymptomatic hypotonic, euvolemic hyponatremia you can treat initially with free water fluid restriction (< 1 liter/day) and treat any underlying cause. Normal saline can be added if needed.
  - » For hypotonic, hypervolemic hyponatremia treatment is fluid restriction to < 1 liter / day and diuretic therapy (if no contraindications).

Practical Pearls:

- In asymptomatic patients being treated for hyponatremia it is a good idea to monitor the Na level twice a day or more so that you can monitor the rate of correction more closely. Patients with symptomatic hyponatremia should probably get more frequent monitoring, especially those on hypertonic saline.
- In asymptomatic hyponatremia, the correction rate should not be more than 0.5 mEq/L/hr.
- In a patient with hyperglycemia, remember to correct the Na. For every increase in glucose of 100mg/dL above 200, the Na falls by 1.6.

Hypernatremia:

- Common causes of hypernatremia in the hospital include: severe dehydration, impaired thirst mechanism, diarrhea, diabetes insipidus, DKA, osmotic diuresis.
- History and exam should be done with a focus on volume status, review of medications and any history of diarrhea and diabetes.
- It is essential to check urine volume and osmolality as this will help determine whether the hypernatremia is from renal or non-renal causes.
- In non-renal causes of hypernatremia the kidneys will produce maximally concentrated urine with low urine volume and high urine osm (usually > 700 mosm/kg).
- In renal causes of hypernatremia such as diabetes insipidus, you should see dilute urine with a serum osm usually < 250 mosm/kg.
- Treatment of hypernatremia:
  - » Increase po (by mouth) free water intake. If patient is npo (nothing by mouth) but has a nasogastric tube (NGT) you can give free water via NGT usually tid (3 times a day). Otherwise you can also treat with D5W or ½ NS IV fluids.
  - » The amount of fluid to be replaced and given can be calculated by using the following formula:
    Water deficit (L) = Current TBW x [(plasma Na – 140) / 140]
    Note: TBW = 0.6 x weight in kg TBW is total body water
  - » This calculated water deficit should be corrected <u>slowly</u> over 48-72 hours sinceoverly rapid correction of Na can lead to central pontine myelinolysis. Goal correction rate should be < 0.5 mmol/L/hr (< 12 mmol/L over first 24 hours).

Shortness of breath (dyspnea):

- Being called for shortness of breath is quite common on the wards. The important thing is to not panic and consider the differential diagnosis.
- The most common causes of shortness of breath on the medical wards are COPD/ asthma flare, CHF exacerbation, pneumonia, PE, MI, anxiety and pneumothorax. The following is a step wise approach on the management of a patient with dyspnea.
- Check the vitals, temperature, pulse ox and take a brief history (ask about any associated chest pain, cough, fevers, chills, recent procedures/ central lines, calf pain/ swelling, as well as nature of the dyspnea). Examine the patient with special attention to the lung and cardiac exam. Other important things to look for on exam would be any evidence of JVD, edema, use of accessory muscles and calf swelling/ pain (for DVT).
- Quickly skim the chart to see if the patient has a history of COPD, asthma, CHF, pneumonia or MI. Also, check if any recent invasive procedures were done (central line placement or thoracentesis) since this may be complicated by a pneumothorax.
- If the patient is hypoxic you should do an ABG (arterial blood gas).
- If the patient is wheezing and has a history of COPD give a stat nebulizer treatment (Atrovent/Albuterol neb tx x 1 stat). Note that albuterol can raise the heart rate.

- If the patient has a history of CHF and you hear crackles in the lungs give Lasix 40mg –80mg IV x 1 (caution in renal patients and in patients with low BP and low K). Also hold their IVF if they are on any.
- If the patient is having chest pain, then get a stat EKG. If cardiac chest pain is suspected then give a sublingual NTG (nitroglycerin) and morphine (2mg IV) if the BP allows. Aspirin should also be given. In some patients (i.e. diabetics) without a clear etiology of dyspnea an EKG should be done to rule out MI even in the absence of chest pain. If cardiac chest pain is suspected please refer to section on chest pain in this book for further management.
- If the patient has a fever, cough and rales this should raise the suspicion for pneumonia and you should start antibiotic therapy, get blood cultures and get stat CXR.
- In a patient with acute SOB/ hypoxia, tachycardia, and a clear lung exam you need to rule out a pulmonary embolism (PE). ABG will often demonstrate an increased A-a gradient and serum d-dimers are almost always elevated. You can consider doing urgent LE dopplers (especially if there is asymmetrical calf pain/ edema) or get a spiral CT or V/Q scan to rule out PE. Depending on the clinical suspicion for PE one must consider empirically starting anti-coagulation therapy if there are no contraindications. Note: For a spiral CT to rule our PE you will need contrast so make sure the patient has normal renal function, is not allergic to IV contrast and also is not pregnant.

- If the patient recently had an invasive procedure such as a central line placement or thoracentesis and is now acutely short of breath you need to rule out a pneumothorax. Check for distended neck veins, decreased breath sounds and hyper-resonance. Order stat chest X-ray. If a pneumo-thorax is present then the patient will need a chest tube or needle decompression.

Practical Pearls:

- In a hypoxic patient you should give supplemental oxygen to maintain a pulse ox >90-92% (PaO2 > 60) because below this number there is a dramatic decline in oxygenation to the tissues.
- In patients that are hypoxic (pulse ox < 90%) or patients with an unclear etiology of dyspnea you should definitely get an ABG, stat CXR and EKG.
- Supplemental oxygen can be given via nasal can-nula, venturi mask, or by non-rebreather mask. 1 L/minute of nasal cannula is equivalent to about 24% FiO2. Each additional liter of oxygen increases the FiO2 by approximately 3-4%. Therefore, a patient on 3 L of oxygen via nasal cannula should be getting about 30-32% FiO2.
- Venturi masks allow for more precise oxygen administration than nasal cannula and therefore in a patient that is hypoxic on nasal cannula, you should switch to a venturi mask. Venturi masks come in 24%, 28% 31%, 35%, 40% and 50% FiO2.
- If a patient is hypoxic on 50% venturi mask then you can try a non-rebreather mask which can give up to 80-90% oxygen.

- Common indications for intubation include hypoxia despite oxygen therapy, hypercapnea, respiratory muscle fatigue, severe acid base disorders, airway protection and acute respiratory decompensation. Refer to the ICU section for further details on mechanical ventilation.
- It is very important to know that when you increase oxygen in a hypoxic patient you should follow up with an ABG since increasing the O2 can lead to CO2 retention and hypercapnia which can be dangerous. This is especially common in patients with COPD/ asthma.

Chest Pain:

- Chest pain is a frequently encountered problem especially on telemetry. As an intern it can be easy to get nervous during the first few times but with some experience you'll see it's usually quite straight forward in most cases.
- Common causes of chest pain include angina, MI, heartburn/ reflux, PE, pericarditis, pneumonia, pleural effusion, musculoskeletal (costochondritis), pleurisy, aortic dissection, pneumtothorax.
- To save time, ask the nurse to start doing an EKG and to get a set of vital signs while you arrive.
- Examine the patient quickly and take a brief history of the chest pain while the EKG is being done. Check the vital signs and a pulse ox. Examine the heart and lungs and also check for any costochondral tenderness.
- Get an idea of the quality and character of the chest pain: ask the patient to quantify the pain from 0-10 (this will help gauge improvement), if there is any radiation of the pain to the neck or down the arm (suggests cardiac chest pain) or to the back (suggests aortic dissection) and if any associated nausea/ vomiting/ diaphoresis. Also ask if the chest pain is pleuritic in nature (suggests PE, pericarditis, pleurisy, pneumonia, or PTX) and if there is any associated dyspnea or cough.
- If you suspect cardiac chest pain and the BP is normal then give a sublingual NTG (nitroglycerin) x 1 and also an aspirin 325 mg to chew. Reassess the BP minutes after the NTG is given. You can give additional NTG after few minutes. Note: It is common for the patient to get a headache after NTG.
- You can also give morphine 2 mg IV x 1 or 2. Morphine may also lower the blood pressure slightly

since it also has vasodilator properties so monitor BP carefully.

- If there are no contraindications, then you should also give metoprolol 2.5-5.0 IV to slow down the heart rate (goal HR about 60 bpm) to decrease the workload on the heart. Make sure the patient is not bradycardic or in heart block and does not have uncontrolled asthma before you give the beta-blocker.
- Any patient with new ST elevation or new LBBB on EKG needs an urgent cardiology evaluation for acute MI and intervention with urgent angioplasty or thrombolytic therapy (if no contra-indications).
- Any patient with new ST depression or dynamic T inversions, also warrants urgent cardiology evaluation and may need to be started on anti-coagulation therapy (heparin/ LMWH +/- IIb/ IIIa inhibitor) if there are no contraindications.
- If ischemia is suspected you should get cardiac enzymes including troponins stat and then q 8 hours.
- Call the attending after the patient is stabilized or if any difficulty in management as he/she should be notified on the status of their patient.

Practical Pearls:

- In a patient with atypical chest pain with a normal exam and EKG you can give Maalox or Mylanta to see if it helps the pain acutely in case it is secondary to heartburn. If chest pain resolved or improves with this then you can add daily proton pump inhibitor therapy.
- In a patient with severe chest pain radiating to the back, very high BP or asymmetric BP in the extremities you should rule out an aortic dissection as well. You can get a stat CXR to see if there is a widened mediastinum or go straight to Echo or CT if your suspicion is high.

Patient that spikes a fever:

- Take a quick history and examine the patient quickly for any obvious sources of infection (ask the patient if they have any cough, urinary symptoms, abdominal pain, diarrhea, headache/ neck stiffness, joint pain/ swelling, rash or any other obvious source of infection).
- Check if the patient had any procedure/ surgery recently or if the patient is getting any blood products (transfusion reaction).
- Do a focused HEENT, lung, heart, abdominal and extremity/ skin exam to look for any obvious source of infection. In elderly bedridden patients look for infected decubitus ulcers as a possible source of infection.
- Order CXR and UA c+s if no obvious source is found on history and exam.
- If the patient has a fever and no recent blood cultures have been done within the last 24- 48 hours then you should also do blood cultures.
- Consider starting empiric antibiotic therapy, <u>especially</u> in immunocompromised or neutropenic patients.
- Can give Tylenol 650 mg po x 1 for fever if it is causing the patient discomfort.
- If fever is high then you can also put the patient on a cooling blanket.
- Common non-infectious causes of fever in the hospital include malignancy (lymphoma), drug fever, connective tissue disorders (SLE). Many inflammatory conditions can also cause fever such as pancreatitis, gout flare but usually these are low grade (< 101 F).

Practical Pearl:

- In a patient on the medical wards or ICU that has a fever you should always assume infection and rule this out first.

Sudden Drop in Hemoglobin:

- Usually a significant drop is > 10% decline in the hemoglobin/ hematocrit (H/H); For example Hgb goes from 10.0 to below 9.0
- Common causes of an <u>acute</u> drop in H/H are dilutional from IVF (intravenous fluids), blood loss (GI, post op bleeding, post cath bleeding/ hematoma or other internal bleeding) and hemolysis.
- The first step is to check the vital signs (including orthostatics) and to do a brief history and exam. Ask of any melena, BRBPR, back pain, abdominal pain, bleeding at IV sites (may suggest DIC or low platelets), recent procedures (cath, surgery).
- Check if the patient is on any anti-coagulation. Ask also about symptoms of severe back pain/ abdominal pain in a patient on anti-coagulation because these could be indicative of a retroperitoneal bleed. Ask about groin pain, swelling, ecchymosis because these could be signs of a bleed into the thigh/ groin area which often occurs post catheterization.
- Send off a repeat CBC stat to confirm decline +/- a Type and screen.
- If you suspect a bleed you should hold anti-coagulation therapy (heparin IV).
- Do a stool guaic in any patient with a drop in H/H to rule out a GI bleed.
- If the patient is orthostatic and guaic positive they need to be NGT (nasogatric tube) lavaged, given blood and IVF resuscitation, transferred to the ICU and urgent GI/ surgery evaluation is warranted. If an UGI bleed is suspected start IV PPI (proton pump inhibitor) therapy. If esophageal varices are considered then also start octreotide.

Practical Pearls:

- Patients on anti-coagulation with a drop in H/H and acute onset of pain (back pain, groin/ thigh pain, abdominal pain) you must rule out a bleed and strongly consider holding anti-coagulation therapy and doing a stat CT scan.
- A common cause of drop in Hgb in the hospital is dilutional from IVF but this is a diagnosis of exclusion.
- An asymptomatic patient with a normal exam and vitals that has a slight drop in H/H you should repeat the CBC again.
- Hemolysis, can be another cause of anemia in the hospital. If suspected, you should order an LDH, haptoglobin, bilirubin, Coombs test and peripheral smear.

Writing for a blood transfusion:

- You need to obtain consent from the patient first.
- Write as: Transfuse 1 or 2 units PRBC's (packed red blood cells).
- In neutropenic patients on chemotherapy you may want to write for leukopoor and irradiated blood products.
- You may choose to premedicate with Tylenol 650 mg po and Benadryl 25 mg po.
- Recheck a CBC 4 hours post transfusion. You should expect the hemoglobin to increase by 1 g/dl for each unit of PRBC's given.

Hypertension:

- Some common secondary causes of hypertension in the hospital include: agitation/ sundowning, pain, anxiety, dyspnea, thyrotoxicosis, iatrogenic (normal saline IVF), and renal artery stenosis.
- Check first if the patient is symptomatic. You should look for signs of target organ disease such as chest pain, pulmonary edema, blurry vision, neurologic symptoms (TIA, stroke symptoms, new onset confusion), interscapular back pain (aortic dissection), hematuria.
- If the patient is <u>symptomatic</u> then you should control the BP urgently with IV medications. Labetolol or nitroprusside are commonly used. If neurologic symptoms are present then do a stat CT of the head. If there is chest pain do an EKG and cardiac enzymes. If the patient is having severe CP radiating to the back, interscapular pain or if there is a significant BP differential in both extremities then you should also rule out an aortic dissection.
- If the patient is <u>asymptomatic</u> and the BP is only moderately elevated ask the nurse if the patient is due for any of their anti-HTN meds any time soon, if they are then you can give their medication earlier and monitor.
- The treatment of HTN is dependent on each patient and their comorbities. For example, if the patient has a history of diabetes and their renal function is normal then an ace inhibitor should be given. Remember to avoid ACE inhibitors if the patient is pregnant, has a history of angioedema, is hyperkalemic or has moderate renal dysfunction. In a patient with a history of CAD/ MI and HTN a beta blocker would be a good choice as long as they do not have any contraindications such as asthma or bradycardia/ heart block.

- Also keep in mind, when you administer a anti-HTN medication that you are aware of what other medications the patient has received during the day for HTN. For instance, if a patient is on a beta-blocker already and has received their daily dose, you do not want to give another order of another beta blocker. You can increase the dose of the one they are taking as long as there are no other contraindications. Likewise, if a patient is on a beta blocker you may not want to give certain medications such as verapamil or diltiazem since these calcium channel blockers can potentiate heart rate lowering.
- In a patient that has symptomatic HTN or hypertensive urgency, it is best to lower the BP with IV medications. Common IV medications to lower BP in hypertensive urgency are again Labetolol or nitroprusside. When patients are on IV drip medications for hypertensive urgency, they do need to be in an ICU setting since BP needs to be continuously monitored. Remember that when lowering BP acutely in a hypertensive patient your goal is to lower the mean arterial pressure (MAP) by 20-25% and not necessarily to completely normalize the BP. Rapid normalization of BP in this setting can result in cerebral hypoperfusion and stroke.

Practical Pearls:

- When on call you are usually covering a vast number of patients and don't have time to learn the
  patient's whole medical history. I personally like
  to use amlodipine 5mg po x 1, in an adult patient
  that has mild-moderate asymptomatic HTN since
  there are really no major contraindications from
  a comorbidity standpoint. You can certainly use
  another ant-HTN medication but that would require
  you to know more about the patient. For example,
  if you wanted to use a beta-blocker you must be
  sure the patient does not have a history of severe
  asthma, bradycardia or heart block. To use an ace
  inhibitor or ARB you would need to make sure that
  the patient does not have significant renal impairment, is not pregnant and does not have a history
  of angioedema.

Nausea and Vomiting:

- Examine the patient to rule out other causes of nausea and vomiting (chest pain/ abdominal pain/ uremia/bowel obstruction / headache (migraine)/ medications (opiods, chemotherapy), etc.
- Any underlying cause should be addressed if found.
- Treatment::
  - » Trimethobenzamide (Tigan) 200 mg IM/ PR or 250 mg po
  - » Prochlorperazine: 5-10mg po q 6-8 hours (max is 40 mg/day)
  - » Promethazine (Phenergan) 12.5-25 mg PO/IM/ PR
  - » Ondansetron 32 mg IV infused over 15 minutes, or can give 8 mg po x 1 (this medication is often used in chemotherapy associated nausea)

Practical Pearl:

- Keep in mind that it may not be wise to give a patient that is vomiting oral (po) meds and it is not wise to give a patient on anti-coagulation therapy with heparin or coumadin IM (intra-muscular) shots.

Anticoagulation Therapy:

PTT adjustment:

- It is very important to keep in mind that different hospitals use different reagents and instruments to calculate PTT. This has major implications on adjusting heparin drips. You should find out if your hospital has a heparin protocol and find out how PTT adjustments are done based on their laboratory. For example at some hospitals a PTT of 45-70 is considered therapeutic where as at another hospital normal may be 60-90.

- The following is an example of a heparin sliding scale (remember this may vary at your institution):

- **PTT < 35** : bolus about 40 units/kg and increase drip by 2.0 units per kg (example 70 kg male bolus 2500 and increase drip by about 150 units/hr); Check PTT in 6 hours.

- **PTT 35-45:** increase drip by 150 – 200 units/ hr (if the patient is large then may give a bolus of 1000-2000 units also); Check PTT in 6 hours.

- **PTT 45-60:** Increase drip by 100- 150 units/hr; Check PTT in 6 hours.

- **PTT 60-90:** Maintain at current rate; Recheck PTT in AM

- **PTT 90-100:** Decrease by 100 units/hr; Check PTT in 6 hours.

- **PTT 101-150:** Decrease drip by 150 units/ hr; Check PTT in 6 hours.

- **PTT >150:** Hold for 1 hour and decrease by 150 units/ hr; Check PTT in 6 hours.

- **PTT > 200:** Hold for 2 hours and decrease by 200 units/hr; Check PTT in 6 hours.

Writing an order for heparin IV:

- Heparin 25,000 units in 500 cc's D5W. Initial bolus is given as 60-80 units/kg with infusion of 14-18 units/kg. Heparin is weight adjusted and thus larger patients will require a higher bolus and infusion dose.
- Occasionally, for acute coronary syndrome or unstable angina the goal PTT some cardiologists prefer is 50-70 and they may prefer to therefore bolus at 60 units/ kg with an infusion rate of 16 units/ hr.

Practical Pearls:

- Anytime you are adjusting heparin always re-check a PTT 6 hours post change. The only time you don't check 6 hours later is if you are maintaining it, then you check in the AM.
- All patients in the hospital on heparin need CBC's and PTT's daily and all patients in the hospital on coumadin need CBC and PT/INR daily.
- In a patient that needs reversal of heparin rapidly, protamine can be given.

Dosing Coumadin:

- When dosing coumadin always remember that the dose of coumadin you give today will not reflect on the INR until 2-3 days later. Therefore, always check the INR and the prior doses of coumadin that the patient has received over the last 3 days and dose accordingly.
- When starting a patient on coumadin for the first time we usually start with coumadin 5mg a day. Any patient on the wards that is on coumadin must have a PT/INR and CBC daily, and you should dose the coumadin only after you have the INR for that day.

- Since it takes about 3 days for the coumadin to reach a therapeutic range we usually have a patient on heparin until the INR is therapeutic.
- Also, since it takes a few days for coumadin to increase the INR you must be patient during the first 2-3 days and not be over aggressive when you see a sub-therapeutic INR since it may go up dramatically after a few days.

Practical Pearls:

- Remember any patient on anti-coagulation with new onset pain in the back, abdomen, extremity, severe headache, etc always consider a bleed. If a bleed is suspected you should hold the anti-coagulation, get a stat CBC and a stat CT. You may need to reverse the anti-coagulation if active bleeding is found. If a bleed is less likely you may still want to get a stat CBC, to make sure there is no drop in H/H. If the H/H has dropped significantly, then you need to hold anti-coagulation and get a stat CT. Never get a stat CBC in a suspected CNS bleed though, go straight to CT scan since it only takes minimal bleeding in the CNS to cause serious harm.
- In patients on Coumadin with bleeding where the effect of Coumadin needs to be reversed rapidly you can give FFP (fresh frozen plasma) and vitamin K.

Insomnia/ Sleeping Pills:

- Insomnia is a frequent problem patients have in the hospital and can be from multiple reasons such as a stress/ anxiety, excess noise (monitors, alarms), disruptive roommate, pain, etc.
- Several medications are often used to help a patient sleep in the hospital:
  - » Zolpidem (Ambien): 5 mg po x 1 (caution in patients with respiratory/ liver impairment)
  - » Estazolam (Prosom): 1mg po x 1 (caution use in patients with respiratory, liver or kidney impairment)
  - » Ramelteon (Rozarem): 8mg po x 1 (caution in liver disease and severe COPD and contraindicated if patient is on fluvoxamine)
  - » Benadryl 25 mg po x 1 (caution anti-cholinergic side effects– urinary retention, tachycardia, etc.)

Practical Pearl:

- Insomnia medications may cause delirium in elderly patients.

Pain control:

- You should always examine the patient to see what is causing the pain (abdominal pain, chest pain, back pain, bone pain, severe headache) and address the underlying cause first.
- Treatment depends on the comorbidities and severity of the pain.
- Mild Pain:
  - » Tylenol 650 mg po
  - » Ibuprofen 400-800 mg (be very cautious with nsaids in patients with renal insufficiency, CHF or on anti-coagulation or history of PUD).
- Moderate Pain:
  - » Percocet 1 tab po q 6-8 hours prn pain
  - » Vicodin 1 tab po q 6-8 hours prn pain
  - » Demerol 70 mg SC/ IM (usually given with vistaril 25 mg SC/ IM)
- Severe Pain:
  - » Morphine 2mg IV q 6 hours
  - » Dilaudid 1-2 mg IV / SC q 6 hrs prn pain (Note: it is not wise to give patients on anti-coagulation IM shots)

Practical Pearl:

- Dilaudid may be slightly safer than Demerol and morphine in patients with renal impairment.

Constipation:

- There are many different causes of constipation in the hospital and they should be investigated in a patient with constipation.
- Some of these include medications (opiods, calcium channel blockers, iron, anti-cholinergic meds), obstruction/ ileus, electrolyte disturbances (hypercalcemia, hypokalemia), hypothyroid, diabetes and immobilization.
- Symptoms of an obstruction or ileus can include abdominal pain, distension, nausea, vomiting, decreased flatus. If this is suspected get an urgent flat and upright X-ray and consider placing an NGT (nasogastric tube) and making the patient NPO (nothing by mouth).
- If there is no obstruction suspected then you can treat with medications. There are many different laxatives or enemas to choose from. Note: I recommend choosing one and seeing if it works before starting multiple agents at the same time.
- Commonly used medications for constipation:
  - » Docusate sodium (Colace) 100mg po bid (stool softener/ laxative)
  - » Senna (senokot) 2 tabs po x 1 (stool softener/ laxative)
  - » Fleets enema x 1 (enema)
  - » MOM (mild of magnesia) 30 cc po x 1(laxative)
  - » Cascara 5cc's po x 1 (laxative)
  - » Lactulose 30 cc po x 1 (laxative)

Practical Pearl:

- Avoid using milk of magnesia (MOM) in patients with renal impairment since they often retain magnesium.
- Be sure to rule out bowel obstruction/ ileus before giving laxatives.
- Spend a little extra time addressing this at admission otherwise you may spend a lot of time regretting it days later when you have to manually disimpact !

Diarrhea:

- Some common causes of diarrhea in the hospital are medications (stool softeners, laxatives, colonoscopy bowel preps, MOM, colchicine, neutral-phos), GI bleeding/ ischemic colitis (blood is a catharctic), IBD, gastroenteritis/ colitis and infections (such as C. diff from antibiotic use).
- Get a brief history and examine the patient. See if there is any abdominal pain, fever, blood in the stool and have the nurse check vitals including orthostatics. See if there is any history of IBD, IBS, gastroenteritis.
- Check to see if the patient received any medications that could cause diarrhea such as the meds mentioned above.
- Rarely, an obstruction can actually cause diarrhea (distal to obstruction) so see if there is any signs or symptoms of obstruction (abdominal pain, distension, nausea, vomiting). If there is then get a stat flat and upright of the abdomen to confirm this.
- If the patient is or has been on antibiotic therapy recently that should raise the suspicion of C. difficile infection and stool should be sent off for C. diff toxin. If C. diff is suspected you should also empirically start treatment with either Metronidazole or po Vancomycin.
- If the patient has symptoms suggestive of gastroenteritis such as fever, abdominal pain, and diarrhea you should also send stool cultures and stool WBC and consider empiric therapy for certain infections.
- If the patient is having moderate-severe diarrhea they can become very dehydrated and develop electrolyte disturbances. Adequate IVF hydration with electrolyte supplementation is often needed.

- If a patient is having mod-severe diarrhea medications such as Immodium or Lomotil may be considered if there are no contraindications. Keep in mind however, that if you suspect an infectious cause to the diarrhea these medications may delay eradication of the infection.

Delirium/ Agitation/ Sundowing:

- Examine the patient first to rule out secondary causes of delirium which include hypoxia, infection, medications, TIA/stroke, withdrawal syndrome, metabolic causes- hyper/hypoglycemia, hyponatremia, etc.
- Check vitals, temperature, pulse ox and obtain a brief history (if possible) and examine the patient including a neurologic exam for any gross abnormalities. In a combative patient this may be difficult but should be done.
- In a patient on insulin, diabetes medications or with poor po intake you should also do an accu-check to make sure the delirium is not secondary to hypoglycemia.
- Check recent blood work results to make sure no other metabolic abnormalities are present (hyponatremia, liver failure, acute renal failure, etc).
- Medications that commonly cause delirium are narcotics, steroids, benzodiazepines, sleeping meds and anti-cholinergic meds.
- If no obvious cause is found, then you can try risperidol 1mg po x 1 if the patient is able to take po.
- If not able to take po then may need to give Haldol. Start at low dose of 1-2mg IM. Can give an additional 1-2 mg more if needed.
- If the patient is a danger to themselves or others then you may need restraints though this should be a last resort.

Practical Pearl:

- In a combative and agitated patient it is often difficult to have them take a po medication and IM (intramuscular) meds may be better.

Patient that fell:

- Get a good, accurate history. Falls are often secondary to loss of footing or slipping.
- It is important, however, to rule out other secondary causes (syncope, arrythmia, vasovagal, CVA/TIA, orthostasis, delirium). A thorough exam including a neurologic exam, cardiac exam, vitals with orthostatics, and inspection for any trauma (bruises/ lacerations) should be done. EKG and monitor should be placed if arrhythmia is suspected.
- Ask the patient if there is any pain anywhere (hip/ back/ribs/extremities/ headache) and if they hit their head. If there is any musculoskeletal pain or signs of trauma then get x-rays of the area to rule out a fracture or in some cases CT to rule out a hemorrhage (ie: headache after a fall).
- Also check to see if the patient is on anti-coagulation.
- Any patient on anti-coagulation with acute pain anywhere after trauma needs imaging (CT) of that area to rule out a bleed. For example, a patient with a severe headache after falling down should get a stat head CT to rule out a bleed.
- Document clearly the details of the fall and your exam. Ask the nurse to put bed rails up and write in orders "fall precautions" if the patient is at danger of falling again.

Seizure:

- Common causes of seizures in the hospital are alcohol withdrawal, hypoglycemia, infection (meningitis, abscess), CVA/ hemorrhage, electrolyte disorders (hyponatremia), medications, anoxia, uremia, drug overdose, malignancy/ mets
- In a patient that is having a seizure you must secure an airway and maintain circulation. Thiamine (100mg IV) followed by glucose (50ml of 50% dextrose) should also be considered.
- Parenteral medications such as lorazepam or diazepam are given acutely to control seizure activity if the patient is actively seizing.
- Patient's history should be reviewed to look for things such as alcohol or drug abuse, signs of infection/ meningitis, history of diabetes or malignancy and the medication list should be reviewed. You should also do a stat accu-check, especially if the patient is on medication for diabetes. Any recent labs should also be checked.
- Once the patient is stabilized, blood work should be sent off including electrolytes, glucose, CBC, BUN/ creatinine, anti-seizure drug levels and tox screens (if applicable).
- If no obvious etiology is found, you should also do a stat CT of the head to rule out malignancy, abscess, bleed, stroke, or mass. If you suspect CNS infection and a head CT is negative then you should do a lumbar puncture to rule out meningitis.
- Phenytoin (dilantin) is commonly used for maintenance anti-convulsant therapy once acute activity is controlled with a benzodiazepine. Dosage and instructions on writing for phenytoin can be found in the chapter on ICU meds and drips.

Elevated blood sugar:

- Some common causes of hyperglycemia in the hospital include uncontrolled diabetes, DKA, steroids, stress response and iatrogenic (D5 IVF).
- For an elevated blood sugar, make sure the patient is not a Type 1 diabetic in DKA; signs and symptoms of DKA include confusion, nausea, vomiting, abdominal pain, polyuria, polydipsia and high anion gap metabolic acidosis.
- If DKA is suspected then you need to get a stat metabolic profile (to check the anion gap), serum acetone level, ABG and UA (check for ketones). You should start aggressive IVF hydration, insulin drip, electrolyte supplementation and transfer to the ICU.
- If asymptomatic hyperglycemia and you do not suspect DKA, then you can check if the patient is simply due for their diabetes medication soon and can give it a little earlier. Otherwise give SQ insulin based on a sliding scale (see below).
- Also look for iatrogenic causes and check if the patient is on D5 IVF or on steroids.
- In a patient with asymptomatic uncontrolled hyperglycemia it is still a good idea to check a basic metabolic profile (+/- serum acetone level) to make sure they do not have a high anion gap metabolic acidosis.

- Based on the glucose, insulin can be given as follows:
- Insulin Sliding Scale (ISS)
- *Blood glucose:* *Insulin units:*
    - » 200-249   2 units
    - » 250-299   4 units
    - » 300-349   6 units
    - » 350-400   8 units

    *Accu-checks q AC and hs, If > 400 or < 60 then call house officer.

    Note: This is a commonly used ISS order. It is rather conservative and some physicians may choose to be more aggressive).

Practical Pearls:

- When admitting a patient with a history of diabetes or if starting steroids on a patient you should write for accu-checks q AC and hs and write an insulin sliding scale order.
- Oral diabetes medications are often held at admission for multiple reasons. Patients may be suddenly made npo for a test, may have abnormal renal function, certain medications/ antibiotics interact with sulfonylureas and potentiate their toxicity or the patient may be going for imaging studies that require contrast. If the medication is being held it is even more important to monitor the blood sugar regularly.
- Before giving an order for insulin over the phone for a patient with mild-moderate hyperglycemia make sure they are not on a oral hypoglycemic agent for diabetes. If they are on a oral hypoglycemic check if they are due to get the medication soon since this may affect the amount of insulin you need to give.

Pronouncing a DNR patient dead:

- Pronouncing a patient dead is emotionally a difficult thing to do as a house officer, especially in the beginning.
- Confirm that there is no pulse, heart beat on auscultation and no spontaneous respirations or movements.
- Confirm that the pupils are fixed and dilated and that there is no response to noxious stimuli (ie: sternal rub)
- Sometimes, it is also a good idea to have a nurse print out a rhythm strip showing asystole for documentation in the chart.
- Once you have done this, write a note in the chart stating all the above and fill out the paperwork given to you by the nurse.
- Always <u>call the attending first</u>, not the family. It should be the attending physician that gets in touch with the family since they usually know the patient and family best. Occasionally an attending may tell you to do this. Be sympathetic to the family and express your sorrow. State law also may require you to ask if an autopsy is wanted by the family.

Decreased urine output:

- Make sure the patient is not an ESRD/dialysis patient.
- If the patient has a foley catheter ask the nurse to make sure it is not clotted by flushing it.
- Make sure the patient is not obstructed (elderly man with BPH and no foley). You may need to insert a foley first, if there is good urine output then it is probably secondary to obstruction. In that case, leave the foley in and treat the underlying cause of the obstruction.
- Another common cause of decreased urine output in the hospital is dehydration/ volume depletion. Examine the patient and their labs to see if they appear volume depleted. If they appear to by dry then give a fluid challenge (500 cc NS bolus) and monitor to see if there is any increase in urine output.
- Acute renal failure can give oliguria or anuria and you should check a basic metabolic profile/ creatinine in these patients to rule out acute renal failure.
- Adequate urine output is about 0.5cc/kg/hr (about 35cc/hr)

Practical Pearl:
- Be cautious in giving IVF challenge in a patient with a history CHF or renal failure.

Hypotension:

- Evaluate the patient for possible causes of hypotension. Medications, sepsis, severe dehydration (vomiting, diarrhea), MI, PE, shock, tamponade, arrhythmia, blood loss, adrenal insufficiency are some common causes of hypotension in the hospital.

- Check to see if the patient is symptomatic (dizzy, lightheaded) and check orthostatics. Try to figure out the cause of the hypotension by history and exam. For example does the patient have fever/ infection (sepsis), was there any recent increase in BP medication dose (iatrogenic), is there any chest pain or SOB (MI or PE), are there any palpitations (arrhythmia), is there any abdominal pain/ melena/ BRBPR (GI bleed), are they on anti-coagulation, did the patient have any recent procedures or surgery (r/o bleed). If the patient had a recent MI then hypotension can also be from tamponade, arrhythmia, or papillary muscle rupture.

- Bolus 250 or 500 cc of Normal Saline stat to bring up the BP. This may need to be repeated. If the BP is not responding to IVF boluses or if the patient can not tolerate the IVF (CHF, ESRD) then you may need to start IV pressors. Be careful giving excessive fluids in a pt with CHF or ESRD.

- Vasoconstrictors that can by used are dopamine, levophed, neo-synephrine. (see ICU section on how to write for these medications)

- Treat the underlying cause while hemodynamically stabilizing the patient. For example in septic shock start antibiotic therapy and send off blood cultures.

DVT prophylaxis: (For non-surgical patients)

- Any patient that is not ambulating/ bedridden in the hospital should probably be on DVT prophylaxis unless contraindicated:
- Options for DVT prophylaxis:
    1. Heparin 5,000 units <u>SC</u> bid-tid for DVT prophylaxis
    2. Enoxaparin (Lovenox) 40mg SC q day.
    3. Dalteparin (Fragmin) 5,000 units SC q day.
- If the patient has contra-indications to anti-coagulation then can use sequential compression boots or stockings.

Practical Pearl:

- If using compression boots make sure that the patient has not been bedridden for more than 1-2 days because in that case you may want to get LE dopplers to rule out a DVT before you apply compression boots. If a DVT has already formed compression boots may cause more problems by dislodging the clot.

Writing Medial Orders:

- *Mnemonic: (ADCVAANDIML)*

Admit to: Service or team name (house officer's name and pager #)

Diagnosis: (examples would be CHF exacerbation, Pneumonia, PE)

Condition: (stable, fair, grave)

Vitals: q shift (as per routine) or q 6 hours depending on the patient

Activity: (depends on each patient/ case): examples are bed rest, OOB (out of bed) to chair, as tolerated.

Allergies: If no medication allergies then write NKDA (no known drug allergies)

Nursing: special instructions for the nurses; this depends on each case and patient (see below)

Diet: (see below)

IV: hep-lock or IVF (Examples: NS at 100 cc's /hr or D5 ½ NS at 75cc's /hr)

Meds: (see below)

Labs:

Here is a brief synopsis of each order:

Admit to: This is where you would write the name of the service the patient is being admitted to and the name of the physician/ house officer responsible for the patient's care.

Diagnosis: This is where you would write the admitting diagnosis for the patient. For example CHF exacerbation, pneumonia, etc.

Condition: This is where you would write the general condition of the patient at admission. Examples would be stable, fair, guarded, etc.

Vitals: This is where you order the frequency at which you want the nurses to check the patient's vital signs. You can also indicate in this section if you would like to have the pulse ox checked with the vitals. Common examples are check vitals q 6 hours, q 8 hours or q shift. Generally on the wards vitals are done every 8 hours or q shift.

Activity: This is where you would write the level of activity you recommend for the patient. Examples would be OOB to chair, ad lib, strict bed rest. This obviously depends on the patient's condition and diagnosis.

Allergies: List any medication or food allergies that the patient may have here.

Nursing: This is where you would write specific nursing orders for your patient that you want the nurses to check. For example:

- If a patient is a diabetic then you should write for accu-checks qAC and HS
- If the patient has a CHF you should write for I's and O's, daily weights and consider writing for fluid restriction (< 1 liter/day)
- If the patient needs a foley then you can write an order for "insert foley".
- If the patient requires oxygen this is where you can write for it. For example: O2 2 liters NC (nasal cannula), check pulse ox q 6-8 hrs and call house officer if pulse ox < 90%.
- If the patient is at risk for aspiration can write aspiration precautions.
- If patient is admitted with a neurologic disorder you can write for neuro checks q 6 hours or q shift.
- If the patient needs sequential boots or stockings you can write for it here as well.

Diet: This is where you would write the diet that you recommend the patient to be placed on. There are many different diets in the hospital and they are patient dependent. Here are some common diets used in the hospital:

- If the patient has diabetes then write for ADA 1800 or 2000 kcal diet.

- If you have a cardiac patient then write for cardiac diet (CD-3 diet)
- If renal insufficiency write for renal diet (2 grams Na, 2 grams K, 60 kg protein)
- If hypertensive write for low salt diet (< 2 grams sodium a day)
- If the patient is not supposed to eat write NPO.
- If lactose intolerant then write for lactose free diet.
- If no medical problems and no dietary restrictions then write for a regular diet.
- Other diets include dysphagia diet, clear liquids, full liquids, low purine diet.

IV: This is where you would write the type and amount of IVF you want your patient to receive. Examples would be D5 1/2 NS at 75 cc/hr or NS at 100 cc/hr. If the patient does not need IVF then just write IV-lock.

Medications: This is where you would write the medication orders for the patient.

- When writing for certain medications such as BP meds, it is a good idea to write for parameters. This can avoid administration of a medication when it may not be indicated. For example: Enalapril 5 mg po qd (hold if SBP is < 100)
- For certain medications like beta-blockers and certain calcium channel blockers like verapamil and diltiazem you should also write for heart rate parameters. For example: Atenolol 50 mg po qd (hold if SBP is < 100 or if HR < 55).

Labs: This is where you would order the labs that you want on your patient. Specify also when you want them done such as stat or in the AM.

Drawing Blood: (Phlebotomy tubes)

Lavender/ purple top: CBC, ABO type

Blue Top: PT/PTT/INR, fibrinogen

Red top (in some hospitals-Yellow top): chemistries (BMP, CMP), electrolytes, cardiac enzymes, LFT's, amylase, lipase, glucose, thyroid, most serum drug levels, PSA, hepatitis, iron.

Gray top: Lactic acid level (on ice)

Green top: Ammonia, thiamine.

Frequently used formulas:

Creatinine clearance: [(140 – age) x weight (kg) x (0.85 if female)] / 72 x serum creat (mg/dl)

Creatinine clearance: from 24 hour urine studies (urine creat x urine volume ml) / (serum creat x time min)

Anion gap: Na – (Cl + HCO3)

A-a gradient: [713 x FiO2) – (paCO2/0.8)] – PaO2

Serum osmolality = (2 x Na) + (Glucose/ 18) + (BUN/ 2.8)

Fractional Excretion of Sodium (FE$_{Na}$) = (U$_{Na}$ x P$_{Cr}$) / (P$_{Na}$ x U$_{Cr}$) x 100

Mean Arterial Pressure (MAP) = diastolic BP + [(systolic BP- diastolic BP) / 3]

Body water deficit (liters) = [0.6 x weight (kg) x (patient Na- normal Na)] / normal Na

Body surface area (m2) = 0.007184 x (Height in cm)$^{0.725}$ x (Weight in kg)$^{0.425}$

INTENSIVE CARE UNIT:

Ventilator management:

Initiation of ventilation:

- When putting a patient on a ventilator you need to set a few parameters such as mode of ventilation, FiO2 level, respiratory rate (RR) and tidal volume (TV).
- Choose the mode of ventilation (most of the time it will be assist control)
- Setting the FiO2. Initially you should always put the patient on 100% FiO2. However, an ABG should be done shortly after intubation and if oxygenation is adequate the FiO2 should be reduced as much as possible while still maintaining an adequate paO2 of > 60-65 (pulse ox > 90-92%). Too much oxygen (high FiO2) for prolonged period is harmful to the lungs from free radical injury.
- Set the respiratory rate (RR), usually start at 12-14 breaths per minute.
- Set the Tidal volume (TV). We usually start at about 6-8 ml/kg of ideal body weight. Thus, in a 70 kg patient you can set the TV to about 500 cc. Note that this approximation of 6-8 ml/kg is based on ideal body weight and not actual weight. Some intensivists may choose to use higher TV up to 10 ml/kg of ideal body weight but this may increase the risk of barotrauma. Low TV also seems to be beneficial in patients with ARDS.

Commonly used Modes of ventilation:

1. _Continuous mechanical ventilation (CMV):_ This is a mode of ventilation that has a set rate and tidal volume. It does not allow for any spontaneous breathing by the patient. This may be used in patients that cannot really initiate a breath, such as patients in deep coma, paralyzed patients, or during anesthesia. Using this mode in patients capable of spontaneous respiratory efforts could lead to patient-ventilator asynchrony. Therefore this mode of ventilation is not commonly used.

2. _Assist control (AC):_ This is the most common initial mode of ventilation used. It delivers a preset TV every time it senses the patient initiate an inspiratory effort. If the patient does not initiate a breath then the ventilator will deliver a full breath at the back-up respiratory rate and TV that is set on the ventilator. A potential problem with this mode is the possibility of respiratory alkalosis if the patient is tachypneic.

3. _Intermittent mandatory ventilation (IMV):_ IMV is similar to AC except, when the patient takes a breath they only get the TV that they inspire and not the TV set on the ventilator, unlike with AC. If the patient does not take a breath then the ventilator will kick in and provide a preset TV at the preset rate. The main difference here is that with IMV when the patient initiates a breath they get the TV that they breathe, whereas with AC when a breath is initiated the ventilator senses this and delivers a full breath at the preset TV. IMV allows the patient to do some of the work of breathing when they inspire and can help to maintain respiratory muscle function and facilitate weaning. With IMV, pressure support if often added (4-8 cm H2O). Pressure support helps overcome the non-physiologic resistance of the ETT and ventilator circuit.

4. _Continuous Positive Airway Pressure (CPAP):_ Is a mode of weaning that is used when trying to wean a patient off the ventilator. It supplies continuous positive pressure and approximates post-extubation breathing. CPAP also allows the advantage of ventilator alarms to remain on so that if there is low minute ventilation or apnea the alarms will sound. CPAP should only be used in patients that are suitable for a weaning trial.

5. _T-piece weaning:_ This is another mode of weaning used by some centers. Once a patient meets weaning criteria, the ETT is attached to a T-piece where one limb is attached to the vent and the other is left open to allow for exhalation. It offers an accurate approximation of post-extubation breathing but does not allow ventilator alarms to remain active and thus requires continuous close observation.

6. _Positive End Expiratory Pressure (PEEP):_ Is positive pressure that is left in the chest after exhalation to prevent alveoli from collapsing. It is not really a mode of ventilation but more an adjunctive tool used in some patients to prevent atelectasis, offer better V/Q matching and improve oxygenation. Typical PEEP used is 5-15cm H_2O. PEEP seems to be beneficial in ARDS. High levels of PEEP can cause pneumothorax and decreased cardiac output with resultant hypotension/ pulmonary edema. PEEP should also be used with extreme caution in patients that are vulnerable to "auto-PEEP" or stacking of breaths such as COPD and asthma patients since these patients may already be generating PEEP on their own from a prolonged expiratory phase and stacking of breaths.

Weaning parameters:

Minimal weaning criteria on ventilator:
1. FiO2 should be 50% or less on the ventilator.
2. RR/TV ratio< 100 (TV is in liters).
3. Minute ventilation < 10 L/min (MV = RR x TV).
4. PaO2/ FiO2 > 240.
5. TV > 300.

Other non-ventilator factors important for weaning:
1. Patient should have appropriate mental status.
2. Sedation should be off or kept minimal to allow for a fair breathing trial.
3. Patient should be hemodynamically stable.
4. Correct any underlying CHF or bronchospasm.
5. Correct any underlying electrolyte abnormalities (low phos).
6. Minimize secretions since this can contribute to failed weaning.
7. Avoid alkalosis since this can decrease respiratory drive.
8. Make sure ABG is adequate before attempting to wean.
9. Ensure adequate nutrition so the patient has enough strength for breathing trial.
10. Use large ETT.

Adjusting the ventilator:

- When adjusting the ventilator, you must focus on 2 things: oxygenation and pH
- Remember the 3 parameters we set initially on the ventilator: FiO_2, RR and TV.
- Adjusting the FiO_2 will only affect oxygenation, where as adjusting the RR and TV will affect the CO_2 and the pH.
- Your goal FiO_2 should be the minimal amount to maintain adequate oxygenation (PaO_2 >60-65 or pulse ox > 90-92% in most cases).
- Very high FiO_2 concentrations (> 60%) can cause excess oxygen free radical formation which can lead to lung injury. It is therefore important to decrease the FiO_2 to the lowest possible level without compromising oxygenation.
- The RR and TV will affect the CO_2 and pH.
- Remember the following: ↑ *RR or TV = ↓ in CO_2 = ↑ pH*
- Therefore if the patient is acidotic you can increase the RR or TV and this should lower the CO_2 and increase the pH. Likewise, in an alkalotic patient with a low CO_2 you can decrease either the RR or TV and this should cause an increase in CO_2 which in turn causes a decrease in pH. Your main objective is to keep the pH normal (around 7.40).
- When adjusting the RR or TV it is important to not only know what the ventilator is set at but also what the patient is breathing at. For example, most patients are on AC ventilation and therefore the machine may be set at a rate of 12 but the patient could be breathing over the vent at 16 breaths a minute. If this is the case, then increasing the ventilator rate to 14 or 16 will not affect the ABG results. In this case it would be better to increase the TV if you wanted to lower the CO_2 and increase the pH.

Peak and Plateau Pressures:

- The peak pressure is the amount of pressure the ventilator requires to deliver a tidal volume against the airway resistance and lung stiffness. The peak pressure should be < 40 cm H2O to avoid barotrauma.
- The plateau pressure is the pressure applied to the small airways after inspiration. The difference between peak and plateau pressure is the airway resistance.
- Therefore, if both peak and plateau pressures are high, then this suggests decreased lung compliance (pulmonary edema, tension PTX, pleural effusion). If the peak pressure is high but the plateau is normal, then this suggests increased airway resistance. This can be from biting on the endotracheal tube (ETT), secretions, bronchospasm, foreign body, kinked tubing etc.

Practical Pearls:

- When putting a patient on a ventilator you should do a stat CXR to confirm proper positioning of the ETT and do an ABG within an hour of intubation to check the pH, paCO2 and paO2 so that adjustments can be made early on.
- When any change in RR or TV is made on a ventilator you should do a repeat ABG shortly thereafter.
- All patients on ventilators should have daily CXR's to confirm proper placement of the ETT and to make sure there is no pneumothorax (a complication of mechanical ventilation).
- In a patient that is not weaning off the ventilator remember to correct the weaning factors mentioned earlier.

Shock:

4 types of Shock:

1. *Hypovolemic Shock:* Results from decrease in intra-vascular volume that leads to decreased preload and resultant decrease in cardiac output. Common causes of hypovolemic shock include blood loss (hemorrhage, GI bleed), fluid loss from diarrhea, vomiting, burns, and third spacing (pancreatitis, ascites). Treatment is aggressive fluid resuscitation with NS or Ringer's lactate. If it is secondary to blood loss you should also give PRBC's.

2. *Cardiogenic Shock:* Is most commonly seen after an MI and is secondary to "pump failure." Other causes include tamponade, arrythmias, acute septal wall rupture or papillary muscle rupture. Treatment is IVF, vasopressors and inotropes. Dopamine is often used in this setting since it has both vasopressor and inotrope properties. Vasodilators can be considered if the patient is hemodynamically stable since decreasing the afterload will improve LV function. Unfortunately, they are seldomly used because patients in cardiogenic shock are often hypotensive already. If medical therapy fails, other non-pharmacologic therapy should be considered such as IABP (intra-aortic balloon pump) to decrease afterload. Eventually the patient will need the underlying problem corrected (angioplasty, valve repair, etc).

3. *Obstructive Shock:* Is most commonly caused by a massive PE. Treatment is initially aimed at maintaining BP by IVF resuscitation (NS) and vasoconstrictors. The underlying cause should be treated (thrombolytic therapy for massive PE in an unstable patient).

4. *Distributive Shock:* Is secondary to a decrease in systemic vascular resistance and is seen in septic shock, anaphylaxis and neurogenic shock. Treatment is

aimed at correcting the underlying cause (antibiotics for septic shock, epinephrine for anaphylaxis)
and maintaining hemodynamic stability with IVF
resuscitation and vasoconstrictors.

Critical Care Parameters & Formulas:

CI = CO / BSA   (Normal = 2.4-4.0 L/min/m2)
CO = SV x HR   (Normal = 4-6 L/min)
SVR = (MAP- mean RAP) x 80/ CO (Normal SVR = 800-1200 dynes/sec/cm-5)
PVR = (mean PAP- PCWP) x 80/CO (Normal PVR = 120-250 dynes/sec/cm-5)

[CI=cardiac index, CO=cardiac output, BSA= body surface area, SV=stroke volume, HR=heart rate, SVR=systemic vascular resistance, MAP=mean arterial pressure, RAP=right atrial pressure, PVR=pulmonary vascular resistance, PAP=pulmonary artery pressure, PCWP=pulmonary capillary wedge pressure]

Hemodynamic Monitoring & Pulmonary Artery Catheterization:

Variable:	Normal:
RAP (right atrial pressure)	2-6 mmHg
RVP (right ventricular pressure)	17-30/0-6 mmHg
PAP (pulmonary artery pressure)	15-30/5-12 mmHg
PCWP (pulm. capillary wedge pressure)	5-12 mmHg

Hemodynamic patterns in different types of shock:

Type of Shock	RAP	RVP	PAP	PCWP	CI	SVR
Hypovolemic	low	low	low	low	low	high
Cardiogenic	high	high	high	high	low	high
Obstructive	high	high	high	norm/ low	low	high/ norm
Distributive	norm/ low	norm/ low	norm/ low	norm/ low	h/n/l (any)	low

Acid Base Disorders & Formulas:

- ❖ *Metabolic acidosis:* Divided into high anion gap and normal anion gap.
- *High anion gap metabolic acidosis:* "MUDPILES" methanol, uremia, DKA, paraldehyde, INH, lactic acidosis, ethylene glycol/ ethanol, and salicylates.
- *Normal anion gap metabolic acidosis:* diarrhea, RTA, carbonic anhydrase inhibitors.
- If metabolic acidosis is the primary disorder, respiratory alkalosis is the compensation. The expected $PaCO_2 = 1.5 \times [HCO3] + 8 \pm 2$
- Delta/ delta (Δ/Δ) = (change in anion gap) / (change in HCO3)
- If Δ/Δ is < 1 a mixed normal and high AG metabolic acidosis is present. If the Δ/Δ is > 1 this suggests a concomitant metabolic alkalosis.

- ❖ *Metabolic alkalosis:*
- Can be divided into chloride (saline) responsive and chloride (saline) unresponsive. Can differentiate between both by urine chloride (Cl). If urine Cl is < 15 then chloride responsive, if urine Cl is > 15 then chloride unresponsive metabolic alkalosis.
- Most primary metabolic alkalosis disorders are chloride responsive and are from volume contraction caused by vomiting, NGT suction or diuretics.
- Chloride unresponsive metabolic alkalosis can be secondary to mineralcorticoid excess (hyperaldosteronism), Liddle's, Bartter's syndrome, Gitelman's syndrome and Cushing's syndrome.
- If metabolic alkalosis is the primary disorder then respiratory acidosis is the compensation. The expected $PaCO_2 = 40 + 0.7$ (Δ in HCO3)

❖ *Respiratory acidosis:*
- Is often secondary to hypoventilation from respiratory depression, neuromuscular disorders, pulmonary disease (COPD, asthma, fibrosis) or drug overdose.
- If respiratory acidosis is the primary disorder then metabolic alkalosis is the compensation.
- If ↑ $PaCO_2$ by 10mm Hg then pH ↓ by 0.08 in <u>acute</u> respiratory acidosis or by 0.04 in <u>chronic</u> respiratory acidosis.
- If ↑ $PaCO_2$ by 10 then HCO_3 ↑ by 1mmol/L in <u>acute</u> respiratory acidosis and ↑ by 3.5 mmol/L in <u>chronic</u> respiratory acidosis.

❖ *Respiratory alkalosis:*
- Causes include hyperventilation, anxiety, salicylates, high altitude, sepsis, liver failure.
- If respiratory alkalosis is the primary disorder then metabolic acidosis is the compensation.
- If ↓ $PaCO_2$ by 10mm Hg then pH ↑ by 0.08 in <u>acute</u> respiratory alkalosis and 0.04 in chronic respiratory alkalosis.
- If ↓ $PaCO_2$ by 10mm Hg then HCO_3 ↓ by 2.0 mmol/L for <u>acute</u> respiratory alkalosis and ↓ by 4.0-5.0 mmol/L for <u>chronic</u> respiratory alkalosis.

Commonly Used Drips in the MICU:

Medication:	Concentration:	Infusion Rate:	Comments:
Amiodarone (Cordarone)	450mg/250ml of D5W	150mg over 10 minutes then 1mg/min x 6hrs then 0.5mg/min for 18 hrs.	Monitor for hypotension. Not compatible with heparin and bicarb.
Amrinone (Inocor)	200mg/100ml NS or 200mg/200ml NS	Bolus 0.75mg/kg IVP over 2 min, then start at 5µg/kg/min and can titrate up to 10-15 µg/kg/min	May cause thrombocytopenia and hepatotoxicity; contains sulfites, not compatible with lasix and sodium bicarb.
Diltiazem (Cardizem)	125 mg/125ml NS or D5W	Can give 0.25mg/kg bolus and then 5-15 mg/hr	Can cause 2nd or 3rd degree heart block, bradycardia, hypotension; do not give with IV beta blocker
Dobutamine (Dobutrex)	250mg/250ml NS or D5W	Start at 3µg/kg/min and can titrate up to 20 µg/kg/min	Not compatible with alkaline solutions; may cause arrythmias and tachycardia; contains sulfites

Drug	Concentration	Dose	Comments
Dopamine	400mg/500ml or 800mg/500ml of D5W or NS	Start at 3 µg/kg/min and titrate to desired effect.	Will also cause tachy-cardia: not compat with alkaline solutions
Epinephrine (Adrenalin)	5mg/500ml of NS or D5W	Start at 1-4µg/min initially and titrate to effect	Not compatible with alka-line solutions
Heparin	25,000 units/ 500ml NS or D5W	Initial bolus 60-80 units/kg, then infusion rate at 14-18 units/kg/hr	Monitor PTT; In acute over-dose or bleeding can give protamine.
Insulin Regular	50 units/ 250 ml NS or 100 units/ 100ml NS	DKA: Bolus 0.1 units/kg IVP and infuse at 0.1 units/kg/hr	Close monitoring of glu-cose required to avoid hypoglycemia
Isoproterenol (Isuprel)	2mg/500 ml D5W or NS	Start at 2µg/min and can titrate up to 10 µg/min	Not compatible with alka-line solutions; avoid using with epin.
Labetolol (Normodyne)	200mg/200ml D5W or NS	Start at 2mg/min and adjust to BP	Monitor for hypotension, bradycardia; caution in asthma/COPD

73

Drug	Concentration	Dosing	Notes
Lidocaine (Xylocaine)	2gm/500ml D5W or NS	Bolus: 1-1.5 mg/kg IVP Infuse at 1-4 mg/min	Monitor for hypertension, arrythmias, paresthesias and CNS side effects/ confusion
Lorazepam (Ativan)	25mg/250ml D5W or NS	Bolus: 2 mg IVP over 1 min, then infuse at 0.5-1.0 mg/hr	May cause respiratory depression.
Midazolam (Versed)	100mg/250ml D5W or NS	Bolus: 0.05-0.2 mg/kg IVP, then infuse at 0.25-2µg/kg/ min	Use caution in CHF and renal patients; Monitor for hypotension
Milrinone (Primacor)	50mg/250ml D5W or NS	Bolus: 50µg/kg IVP over 10 min and infuse at 0.375-0.75µg/ kg/min	Not compatible with furosemide; Needs adjust-ment in renal impairment
Morphine Sulfate	62.5mg/250ml D5W or NS	Start at 0.5 mg/hr and titrate up	Monitor for respiratory depression
Nitroglycerin (Tridil)	50mg/ 250ml D5W or NS	Start at 50 µg/ min	Monitor for hypotension
Nitroprusside (Nipride)	50mg/250ml D5W only	Start at 0.25 µg/kg/min and titrate to effect up to max of 10µg/kg/min	Monitor for hypotension; Use for shortest duration possible; monitor for cya-nide toxicity; protect from the light.

Norepinephrine (Levophed)	8mg/500ml D5W only	Start at 2μg/min and titrate to effect.	Avoid abrupt withdrawal
Phenylephrine (Neo-synephrine)	10mg/250ml NS or D5W	Start at 10μg/min and titrate to effect	Avoid in severe HTN and bradycardia
Propofol (Diprivan)	1000mg/100ml (premixed)	Start at 5μg/kg/min and titrate up	Can cause respiratory depression, hypotension; monitor triglycerides with prolonged use.
t-PA (Activase)	100mg/100ml SWFI	Bolus: 15mg IVP over 1-2 min, then infuse 50mg over 30 min, then 35 mg over 60 min. (Note: If weight < 70 kg use 15 mg bolus then infuse 0.75mg/kg for 30 min then 0.5mg/kg for 1 hour)	Patient must be on cardiac monitor; total dose should no exceed 100mg; monitor for signs of bleeding

ACLS Protocols:

Bradycardia:

1. Primary survey (ABC's)
2. Secondary survey (oxygen, IV access, EKG, focused history/ exam)
3. If serious signs or symptomatic then can do transcutaneous pacing if available or administer one of the following:
   » atropine (0.5-1 mg)
   » epinephrine (2-10 µg/min)
   » dopamine 5-20 µg/kg/min
4. If asymptomatic then check EKG.
   » If EKG normal then observe and monitor.
   » If EKG shows Type II 2nd degree or CHB then need pacemaker.

Asystole:

1. Primary survey (ABC's) and start CPR
2. Secondary survey (oxygen, IV access, identify rhythm, treat)
3. Treatment includes:
   » Epinephrine 1 IVP (can repeat q 3-5 minutes)
   » Atropine 1 mg IV (can repeat q 3-5 minutes - up to 3 doses)

PEA:

1. Primary survey (ABC's) and start CPR
2. Secondary survey (oxygen, IV access, identify rhythm, treat, look for causes)
3. Most frequent causes of PEA (5 H's and 5 T's)
   » Hypovolemia, Hypoxia, H ion excess (acidosis), Hyper/hypokalemia, Hypothermia
   » Tamponade, Tension PTX, Thrombosis (MI), Thrombus (PE), Tablets (drug OD)
4. Medication therapy:

» Epinephrine 1 mg IVP (can repeat q 3-5 minutes)
» Atropine 1 mg IV (repeat q 3-5 minutes - up to 3 doses)

Ventricular Fibrillation (VF) or Pulseless Ventricular Tachycardia (VT):

1. Primary survey (ABC's, assess rhythm, CPR)
2. If VF or pulseless VT then defibrillate at 360 J if using a monophasic defibrillator (equivalent on a biphasic can vary from 120 – 200 J), and resume CPR. Note: This ACLS guideline of giving only one shock initially was recently revised from the prior protocol of giving 3 shocks.
3. Assess rhythm after shock and check for pulse. If rhythm still shows VF or pulseless VT then administer:
   » Epinephrine 1mg IVP q 3-5 min <u>or</u> vasopressin 40 U IV single dose only
4. Resume CPR, assess rhythm and defibrillate (360 J or biphasic equivalent) if rhythm unchanged.
5. If still in VF or pulseless VT start anti-arrythmic therapy:
   » *Amiodarone:* Initial: 300mg IVP, can repeat another 150 mg IVP in 3-5 min if refractory; max dose 2.2 g IV over 24 hours.
   » *Lidocaine:* Initial: 1-1.5 mg/kg IV; If refractory VF can give additional 0.5-0.75 mg/kg IVP to max of 3 mg/kg.
   » *Magnesium:* 1-2 grams IV for torsades
   » *Procainamide:* 20 mg/min IV infusion (max total 17 mg/kg). (can be considered if refractory to above meds)
6. Reattempt to defibrillate (360 J or biphasic equivalent).
7. Remember to give epinephrine every 3-5 minutes (unless you gave vasopressin). Frequently check the rhythm and pulse and continue CPR.

Unstable and Stable Ventricular Tachycardia (VT):

1. Check to see if the patient is stable or unstable and see if they are symptomatic.
2. If the patient has V-tach with no pulse on exam then see VF/ pulseless V-tach algorithm above.
3. If (+) pulse and unstable VT then prepare for synchronized cardioversion.
4. If (+) pulse and stable VT check if it is mono or polymorphic.
5. Treatment of monomorphic VT:
   » Amiodarone: (150 mg IV over 10 min and repeat if needed)
   » Lidocaine: (0.5- 0.75 mg/kg IVP) can be considered if refractory to amiodarone.
   » Synchronized cardioversion can also be used.
6. Treatment of polymorphic VT or torsades:
   » Magnesium 1-2 grams IV.

Narrow Complex Supraventricular Tachycardias:

1. Assess the patient to see if stable or unstable and review EKG.
2. If unstable then need to prepare for synchronized cardioversion.
3. Check if narrow complex tachycardia is regular or irregular.
4. If irregular this suggests atrial fibrillation, MAT (multifocal atrial tachycardia) or possible atrial flutter and initial therapy if focused on rate control with beta-blockers (ie: metoprolol or atenolol) or diltiazem.
5. If narrow complex tachycardia is regular then can try vagal stimulation (avoid if bruits or history of carotid disease) and can give adenosine 6-12 mg IVP.
6. If the rhythm does not convert and the patient is stable you can use rate control medications such as beta-blockers (metoprolol, atenolol) or diltiazem.

Important Phone Numbers & Extensions in the Hospital:

ER: _____

ICU: _____

Telemetry: _____

Pharmacy: _____

Lab: _____

Clinic: _____

On call room: _____

Cafeteria: _____

X-ray: _____

CT: _____

MRI: _____

U/S: _____

OB: _____

Wards 1: _____

Wards 2: _____

Wards 3: _____

Wards 4: _____

Wards 5: _____

Notes

Notes

Notes